Complex Regional Pain Syndrome

A Beginner's Quick Start Guide to Managing CRPS Through Diet, With Sample Curated Recipes

mf

copyright © 2022 Larry Jamesonn

All rights reserved No part of this book may be reproduced, or stored in a retrieval system, or transmitted in any form or by any means, electronic, mechanical, photocopying, recording, or otherwise, without express written permission of the publisher.

Disclaimer

By reading this disclaimer, you are accepting the terms of the disclaimer in full. If you disagree with this disclaimer, please do not read the guide.

All of the content within this guide is provided for informational and educational purposes only, and should not be accepted as independent medical or other professional advice. The author is not a doctor, physician, nurse, mental health provider, or registered nutritionist/dietician. Therefore, using and reading this guide does not establish any form of a physician-patient relationship.

Always consult with a physician or another qualified health provider with any issues or questions you might have regarding any sort of medical condition. Do not ever disregard any qualified professional medical advice or delay seeking that advice because of anything you have read in this guide. The information in this guide is not intended to be any sort of medical advice and should not be used in lieu of any medical advice by a licensed and qualified medical professional.

The information in this guide has been compiled from a variety of known sources. However, the author cannot attest to or guarantee the accuracy of each source and thus should not be held liable for any errors or omissions.

You acknowledge that the publisher of this guide will not be held liable for any loss or damage of any kind incurred as a result of this guide or the reliance on any information provided within this guide. You acknowledge and agree that you assume all risk and responsibility for any action you undertake in response to the information in this guide.

Using this guide does not guarantee any particular result (e.g., weight loss or a cure). By reading this guide, you acknowledge that there are no guarantees to any specific outcome or results you can expect.

All product names, diet plans, or names used in this guide are for identification purposes only and are the property of their respective owners. The use of these names does not imply endorsement. All other trademarks cited herein are the property of their respective owners.

Where applicable, this guide is not intended to be a substitute for the original work of this diet plan and is, at most, a supplement to the original work for this diet plan and never a direct substitute. This guide is a personal expression of the facts of that diet plan.

Where applicable, persons shown in the cover images are stock photography models and the publisher has obtained the rights to use the images through license agreements with third-party stock image companies.

Table of Contents

Introduction — 7
What Causes Complex Regional Pain Syndrome? — 9
   What are the two types of CRPS? — 10
What Are the Symptoms of Complex Regional Pain Syndrome? — 11
   How is CRPS diagnosed? — 12
What Are the Treatment for CRPS? — 14
   What are the complications of CRPS? — 15
How Can CRPS Be Prevented? — 19
   Who is at risk to get CRPS? — 19
How to Manage CRPS Through Natural Methods and Lifestyle Changes? — 22
Managing Complex Regional Pain Syndrome Through Diet — 25
   Anti-inflammatory Diet — 25
   Foods to Avoid — 27
Sample Recipes — 31
   Vegan Caribbean Bowl — 32
   Baked Flounder — 34
   Salmon with Avocados and Brussels Sprout — 35
   Asian-Themed Macrobiotic Bowl — 38
   Chicken Salad — 40
   Baked Salmon — 41
   Asian Zucchini Salad — 42
   Low FODMAP Burger — 43
   Stir-Fried Cabbage and Apples — 44
   Asparagus and Greens Salad with Tahini and Poppy Seed Dressing — 45
   Stir-Fried Cabbage and Apples — 46
   Roasted Chicken Thighs — 47
   Arugula and Mushroom Salad — 48

Cauliflower and Mushroom Bake	49
Conclusion	**50**
FAQ About Complex Regional Pain Syndrome	**52**
References and Helpful Links	**54**

Introduction

Complex regional pain syndrome, often known as CRPS, is an umbrella term used to describe an excessive amount of pain and inflammation that occurs after an injury to an arm or leg.

The exact cause of CRPS is unknown, but it is believed to be the result of a malfunction in the nervous system. The condition can develop after any type of injury, including a minor injury such as a sprained ankle.

CRPS can result in a wide range of symptoms, including burning pain, swelling, and stiffness in the affected limb. The condition can also cause changes in skin color and temperature, as well as loss of hair and nails.

CRPS is a complex condition that is often difficult to diagnose and treat. There is no cure for CRPS, but early diagnosis and treatment can help to reduce the severity of symptoms.

There are a variety of treatments available for CRPS, including medication, physical therapy, and nerve blocks. Diet is also an important part of managing CRPS.

Certain foods can help to reduce pain and inflammation, while others may worsen symptoms. It is important to work with a healthcare provider to create a diet plan that is right for you.

In this quick start guide, we'll provide in-depth detail about the following:

- What causes complex regional pain syndrome?
- What are the two types of CRPS?
- What are the symptoms of complex regional pain syndrome?
- How is CRPS diagnosed?
- What are the treatments for CRPS?
- What are its complications?
- Who is at risk to get CRPS?
- How to manage CRPS through natural methods and lifestyle changes?
- Managing complex regional pain syndrome through diet

So, let's get started!

What Causes Complex Regional Pain Syndrome?

The exact cause of CRPS is unknown. However, it is believed to be the result of the following:

- *Malfunction in the nervous system:* CRPS is thought to be the result of a malfunction in the nervous system. This can occur after an injury, surgery, or infection.

- *Abnormal inflammatory response:* CRPS is also believed to be the result of an abnormal inflammatory response. This means that the body's immune system is overreacting to an injury or infection.

- *Damage to the blood vessels:* CRPS may also be the result of damage to the blood vessels. This can cause a decrease in blood flow to the affected area and lead to pain, swelling, and other symptoms.

What are the two types of CRPS?

There are two types of CRPS: type 1 and type 2. Both types of CRPS can cause severe pain, swelling, and changes in skin color and temperature.

- *Type 1 CRPS:* Also known as reflex sympathetic dystrophy (RSD), is the most common type of CRPS. It typically develops after an injury or surgery to the arm or leg.
- *Type 2 CRPS:* Also known as causalgia, is less common than type 1 CRPS. It typically develops after an injury to a nerve.

What Are the Symptoms of Complex Regional Pain Syndrome?

Complex regional pain syndrome (CRPS) is a condition that can cause a wide variety of symptoms. Some people may experience constant pain, while others may have episodes of severe pain. Other common symptoms include swelling, stiffness, and changes in skin color or temperature. The symptoms of CRPS can vary from person to person, and they often change over time.

- *Pain:* The pain associated with CRPS is usually described as a burning or prickling sensation. It is often worse at night. The pain may be constant or intermittent and can vary in intensity.
- *Swelling:* Swelling is a common symptom of CRPS. The affected limb may feel larger than usual and the skin may appear tight or shiny.
- *Stiffness:* Stiffness is another common symptom of CRPS. The affected limb may feel stiff and difficult to move.

- *Changes in skin color:* The skin of the affected limb may change color. It may become red, blue, or purple. The skin may also be warm to the touch.
- *Changes in skin temperature:* The skin of the affected limb may feel warm or cold. It may also sweat more than usual.
- *Changes in hair and nails:* The hair and nails on the affected limb may change. The hair may become thin or fall out. The nails may become brittle or discolored.

How is CRPS diagnosed?

No one test can definitively diagnose CRPS, so doctors often rely on a combination of tests and procedures to make a diagnosis. Some of the tests that may be used include imaging studies, nerve conduction studies, and blood tests. If CRPS is suspected, doctors will typically start by trying to rule out other possible causes of the pain.

- *Medical history:* A healthcare provider will take a medical history and ask about your symptoms.
- *Physical examination:* A physical examination will be done to look for signs of CRPS. The affected limb may be swollen, discolored, or warm to the touch.
- *Imaging tests:* Imaging tests, such as x-rays or MRIs, may be done to rule out other conditions.

- ***Blood tests:*** Blood tests may be done to look for inflammatory markers.
- ***Nerve tests:*** Nerve tests, such as nerve conduction studies or electromyography (EMG), may be done to assess the function of the nerves.

What Are the Treatment for CRPS?

Complex regional pain syndrome (CRPS) is a condition that has no cure. There are, however, a variety of treatments available to help lessen the symptoms. Some of these include medications, physical therapy, and surgery. While there is no cure for CRPS, finding the right treatment plan can help improve the quality of life for those living with this condition.

- *Medications:* Medications, such as analgesics, anti-inflammatories, and nerve blockers, may be used to relieve pain.
- *Physical therapy:* Physical therapy may be used to improve range of motion and muscle strength.
- *Occupational therapy:* Occupational therapy may be used to help you learn how to perform activities of daily living with CRPS.
- *Surgery:* Surgery may be an option in some cases. Surgery is typically done to relieve pressure on a nerve or to repair damaged blood vessels.

What are the complications of CRPS?

Complex regional pain syndrome (CRPS) is a debilitating condition that can lead to a variety of complications. These complications can include but are not limited to, chronic pain, loss of ROM, bone loss, depression, anxiety, and sleep disturbances. In some cases, CRPS can even be fatal.

For these reasons, people with CRPS need to seek medical treatment as soon as possible. While there is no cure for CRPS, there are treatments available that can help lessen the symptoms and improve the quality of life.

- *Chronic pain:* The pain is often out of proportion to any injury or underlying condition. In some cases, the pain may be so severe that it interferes with a person's ability to perform activities of daily living.

  Chronic pain is one of the most common complications of CRPS, and it can have a profound impact on a person's quality of life. If you are suffering from chronic pain, it is important to seek treatment so that you can live as normal a life as possible.

- *Muscle weakness:* Muscle weakness is a common complication of complex regional pain syndrome. The condition can cause the muscles to become weak and atrophied, which can lead to difficulty moving the affected limb. In severe cases, it may even be impossible to move the limb at all. Muscle weakness can also make it difficult to perform everyday activities, such as getting dressed or brushing your teeth.

In addition, the condition can cause severe pain, making it difficult to sleep or concentrate. If you are experiencing muscle weakness, it is important to talk to your doctor so that you can receive the treatment you need. There are a variety of treatments available that can help to relieve the symptoms of complex regional pain syndrome. You can experience significant improvements in your quality of life with proper treatment.

- *Joint stiffness and swelling:* Joint stiffness and swelling are both complications of inflammation, which can be a major problem for people with CRPS. Inflammation can lead to further pain and damage to the joints, making it difficult for people with CRPS to move about and perform daily activities. In severe cases, joint stiffness and swelling can lead to joint deformity and disability. There is no cure for CRPS, but treatment focuses on relieving pain and improving quality of life.

- *Loss of range of motion:* One of the most common complications of CRPS is loss of range of motion (ROM). This can occur when the joints in the affected limb become inflamed, making it difficult to move the joint through its full range of motion. Loss of ROM can also occur when the muscles in the affected limb atrophy, or waste away. This can happen if the muscles are not used often enough, or if they are not receiving enough blood flow. In some cases, loss of ROM may be permanent.

If you are experiencing a loss of ROM due to CRPS, it is important to seek medical treatment as soon as possible. Early intervention can help to prevent further damage and improve your chances of recovery.

- *Lymphedema:* One of the possible complications of CRPS is lymphedema, which is a swelling of the soft tissue due to the accumulation of lymph fluid. Lymphedema can occur in any part of the body but is most commonly seen in the arms or legs.

  There are two types of lymphedema: primary and secondary. Primary lymphedema is caused by a dysfunction in the lymphatic system, while secondary lymphedema is caused by damage to the lymphatic vessels. Lymphedema can lead to severe pain, disability, and emotional distress. People with CRPS need to be aware of the potential complications so that they can seek early treatment if necessary.

- *Bone loss:* Bone loss occurs when the body breaks down bone tissue faster than it can rebuild it. This can lead to thinning of the bones and an increased risk of fractures. In severe cases, bone loss can cause the affected limb to become shorter or deformed.

- ***Depression, anxiety, and sleep disturbances:*** CRPS can also lead to complications, such as depression, anxiety, and sleep disturbances. Depression is common in people with chronic pain conditions, and it can be exacerbated by the isolation and stress of living with a debilitating condition. Anxiety can also be triggered by fear of movement and fear of re-injury. Sleep disturbances are another common complication of CRPS, as the pain can make it difficult to fall asleep or stay asleep.

These complications can have a major impact on your quality of life, so it is important to seek treatment if you are experiencing any of them.

How Can CRPS Be Prevented?

There is no sure way to prevent CRPS. However, early diagnosis and treatment may help to improve the outcome.

If you have had an injury or surgery, it is important to follow your healthcare provider's instructions for recovery. This may help to reduce your risk of developing CRPS.

Who is at risk to get CRPS?

While the exact cause of complex regional pain syndrome (CRPS) is unknown, several risk factors have been identified.

- *Age:* CRPS is most likely to develop in adults aged 40-60. This may be because older adults are more likely to experience injuries or diseases that can trigger CRPS. For example, a break or surgery in an older adult is more likely to cause complications such as nerve damage, which can lead to CRPS.

  Additionally, age-related changes in the nervous system may make older adults more susceptible to developing CRPS. Despite this, CRPS can occur at any age, and further research is needed to determine why some people are more susceptible than others.

- *Previous trauma:* CRPS typically occurs after an injury to the arm or leg, and surgery is also a common trigger. It is thought that the initial injury disrupts the normal functioning of the nervous system, which in turn leads to the development of chronic pain.

  In some cases, CRPS may even occur in the absence of an obvious injury or surgery. However, previous trauma is still believed to be a major risk factor. Therefore, anyone who has sustained an injury or undergone surgery should be aware of the potential for developing CRPS.

- *ACE inhibitors:* ACE inhibitors are a type of medication used to treat high blood pressure. They work by relaxing the blood vessels, which lowers blood pressure.

  ACE inhibitors have been linked to an increased risk of developing CRPS. This may be because they can contribute to nerve damage, which can lead to chronic pain. Therefore, people taking ACE inhibitors should be aware of the potential for developing CRPS.

- *Other risk factors:* Other potential risk factors for CRPS include diabetes, smoking, and certain viral infections. However, further research is needed to confirm these risk factors.

People with these risk factors should be aware of the potential for developing CRPS so that they can seek early treatment if necessary.

How to Manage CRPS Through Natural Methods and Lifestyle Changes?

Complex regional pain syndrome (CRPS) is a debilitating condition that can be extremely difficult to manage. While there is no one-size-fits-all approach to managing CRPS, there are several natural methods and lifestyle changes that can help ease symptoms. Some of the most effective strategies include:

- *Exercise:* Exercise is often recommended as a way to improve the range of motion and reduce pain. However, it is essential to start slowly and increase the intensity gradually. Exercise can help to improve CRPS symptoms, but it is important to start slowly and increase the intensity gradually. Otherwise, you may worsen your symptoms or cause more pain.

    If you have CRPS, talk to your doctor before starting an exercise program. They can help you develop a safe and effective plan that meets your needs and goals.

- *Heat and cold therapy:* Heat and cold therapy can help to improve blood circulation and reduce pain. Cold therapy reduces inflammation by constricting blood vessels, while heat therapy dilates blood vessels and increases blood flow. Heat and cold therapy can also be used in combination to provide additional relief.

- *Massage:* Massage is an effective treatment for complex regional pain syndrome (CRPS). Massage therapy is thought to work by reducing inflammation and promoting blood flow to the affected area. This, in turn, helps to relax the muscles and reduce pain. In addition, massage can help to reduce stress and anxiety, which can further contribute to pain relief.

- *Acupuncture:* Acupuncture is a form of Chinese medicine that involves inserting thin needles into the skin. Acupuncture is effective in relieving pain.

- *Yoga:* Yoga is an effective way to manage CRPS symptoms. The gentle stretching and relaxation poses can help improve flexibility, mobility, and overall well-being. If you're not familiar with yoga, consider attending a class at a local studio or finding some yoga videos online.

- *Biofeedback:* Biofeedback is a technique that uses sensors to measure body functions, such as heart rate and muscle tension. The information is then used to help you learn to control these functions.

- *Diet:* Modifying your diet can help improve symptoms of CRPS. Foods that are high in antioxidants, such as fruits and vegetables, may help reduce inflammation and pain. It's also important to drink plenty of water and avoid foods that are high in sugar and processed carbohydrates.

Managing Complex Regional Pain Syndrome Through Diet

There is no one specific diet for people with CRPS. However, eating a healthy diet that includes anti-inflammatory foods may help to reduce pain and inflammation.

Anti-inflammatory Diet

There is growing evidence that anti-inflammatory foods can help to reduce pain and inflammation. People who eat a diet high in these nutrients tend to have lower levels of inflammation.

Additionally, they are also less likely to experience pain. This is thought to be because these nutrients help to reduce oxidative stress and inflammation in the body. As a result, they may be beneficial for people who suffer from CRPS. Anti-inflammatory foods include:

- ***Omega-3 fatty acids:*** Omega-3 fatty acids are a type of unsaturated fat that is found in fish oil. They have anti-inflammatory properties, which makes them effective in reducing the inflammation associated with

CRPS. In addition, omega-3 fatty acids can help to reduce pain levels and improve joint function. As a result, they are an important part of managing CRPS and improving patient outcomes.

Omega-3 fatty acids are found in fish, such as salmon, tuna, and sardines. They are also found in flaxseeds, chia seeds, and walnuts.

- *Turmeric:* Turmeric is a spice that is often used in Indian food. It contains curcumin, which has anti-inflammatory properties.

- *Ginger:* Ginger has been used for centuries as a natural remedy for a variety of ailments. The most well-known benefit of ginger is its ability to relieve nausea, but it is also effective in treating inflammation and pain. It is also a powerful antioxidant, helping to protect cells from damage.

- *Green leafy vegetables:* Green leafy vegetables, such as spinach and kale, are high in vitamins and minerals. They also contain antioxidants that can help to reduce inflammation.

In addition to eating anti-inflammatory foods, it is important to eat a variety of other healthy foods. These include fruits, vegetables, whole grains, and lean protein.

It is also important to stay hydrated by drinking plenty of water.

CRPS can be a debilitating condition. However, some treatments can help to relieve pain and other symptoms. Natural methods and lifestyle changes may also help. Eating a healthy diet that includes anti-inflammatory foods is one way to help reduce pain and inflammation.

Foods to Avoid

There are no specific foods to avoid with CRPS. However, some people find that certain foods trigger their symptoms. These trigger foods may vary from person to person.

- *Sugar:* Sugars are a type of carbohydrate that the body uses for energy. However, too much sugar can lead to a condition called insulin resistance, which is when the body's cells stop responding properly to insulin. This can cause inflammation in the body, as well as a host of other problems such as weight gain, diabetes, and heart disease.

    While it's important to consume some sugar as part of a healthy diet, it's important to be aware of how much sugar you're consuming and to limit your intake to prevent these negative health effects.

- *Refined flours:* Refined flours are made by removing the wheat germ and bran, which contain most of the nutrients. The result is flour that is higher in sugar and lowers in fiber, vitamins, and minerals. This can cause blood sugar levels to spike, leading to inflammation and a host of other health problems.

In addition, refined flours are often bleached with chemicals that can be harmful to the body. For these reasons, it's best to avoid refined flour and choose whole grain alternatives instead.

- *Red meat:* Many people enjoy the taste of red meat and it can be a good source of protein, however, it is also high in saturated fat. Saturated fat is known to trigger inflammation in the body, which can lead to pain, swelling, and other CRPS symptoms. For this reason, it's best to limit your intake of red meat or choose leaner cuts when possible.
- *Processed foods:* Processed foods are foods that have been altered from their natural state. They often contain additives and preservatives that can be harmful to the body. In addition, processed foods are often high in sugar, salt, and unhealthy fats. These ingredients can all trigger inflammation, which can worsen CRPS symptoms. For this reason, it's best to limit your intake of processed foods and choose whole, unprocessed foods instead.
- *Butter:* Butter is a dairy product that is made from the fat and protein in milk. It is a popular ingredient in

many recipes, but it is also high in saturated fat. This type of fat can trigger inflammation, which is a response by the body's immune system.
- *Whole eggs:* Whole eggs are high in cholesterol, and consuming too much cholesterol can trigger inflammation. Additionally, the yolks of eggs contain a substance called lecithin, which can also cause inflammation.
- *Coffee:* Coffee is a popular morning drink, but it can also be a source of anxiety and stress. The caffeine in coffee is a stimulant, which can increase heart rate and blood pressure. This can lead to feelings of anxiousness and agitation.
- *Alcohol:* Alcohol is a known trigger for CRPS symptoms. It can cause inflammation and pain in the body. In addition, alcohol can interfere with medications that are used to treat CRPS. For these reasons, it's best to avoid alcohol or limit your intake if you do drink.
- *Chocolate:* Chocolate contains caffeine. Caffeine is a stimulant and can trigger anxiety and stress. In addition, caffeine can also cause inflammation.

If you suffer from CRPS, it's important to be aware of the foods that may trigger your symptoms. By avoiding these trigger foods, you can help to reduce pain and inflammation. In addition, eating a healthy diet that includes anti-inflammatory foods can also help to manage CRPS symptoms.

Sample Recipes

Vegan Caribbean Bowl

Ingredients:
- 1 cup jasmine rice
- 1 cup coconut milk
- 1 cup broth
- 1 tsp. salt
- 1/4 cup unsweetened dried coconut flakes, shredded
- 4 leaves kale or collard greens, stems removed and sliced thinly
- 1/4 white cabbage, shredded
- 1/2 red bell pepper, julienned
- 1 lime, halved
- 1 tbsp. coconut oil
- 1/2 orange
- Optional: 1-2 tsp. sesame oil
- Optional, choices for garnish: avocado, carrot, cilantro lime, orange, pineapple, and/or scallion, may be combined or not

Marinade:
- 1/2 cup fresh squeezed orange juice
- 1/4 cup soy sauce
- 1 tbsp. jerk seasoning
- 1 tsp. toasted sesame oil (Asian variety)
- tempeh, cubed or sliced (may also use other protein sources if desired)

Instructions:

For the marinade:

1. Mix the marinade ingredients.
2. Throw in the tempeh in the marinade. Let it soak for at least half an hour.
3. In a saucepan, pour in the rice, coconut milk, broth, coconut flakes, and salt.
4. Set to medium-high heat and leave to boil.
5. Lower heat and allow to simmer for about 20 minutes, covered.
6. Once done, turn off the heat and leave the rice for now.
7. In a bowl, put red pepper, kale, and cabbage. Squeeze half a lime over.
8. In a pan placed over medium-high heat, pour in coconut oil.
9. Add the marinated tempeh to the hot oil. Cook until all sides are cooked well.
10. Add a teaspoon or two of sesame oil if desired. Squeeze in half an orange.
11. Remove tempeh from the pan.
12. In a serving bowl, scoop in rice, tempeh, and vegetables.
13. Upon serving, garnish according to your preference.

Baked Flounder

Ingredients:

- 1 lb. flounder, filleted
- 1/4 tsp. salt
- 1 cup halved red grapes
- 1 tbsp. extra-virgin olive oil
- 2 tbsp. parsley, chopped finely
- 1 tbsp. lemon juice
- 1 cup almonds, chopped and toasted
- freshly ground black pepper, to taste

Instructions:

1. Preheat the oven to 375°F.
2. Place fish on a sheet tray. Season with olive oil, salt, and pepper.
3. Combine the almonds, grapes, lemon juice, parsley, 1-1/2 tsp. of olive oil, 1/8 tsp of salt, and black pepper in a bowl.
4. Bake the fish for about 3 minutes.
5. Flip the fish and return it to the oven.
6. Bake for another 3 minutes, or until the fish is starting to flake, while the center is still translucent. Don't overcook.
7. Serve immediately, topped with the grape mixture.

Salmon with Avocados and Brussels Sprout

Ingredients:

- 2 lbs. of salmon filet, divided into 4 pieces
- 1 tsp. ground cumin
- 1 tsp. onion powder
- 1 tsp. paprika powder
- 1/2 tsp. garlic powder
- 1 tsp. chili powder
- Himalayan sea salt
- black pepper, freshly ground

Avocado sauce:

- 2 chopped avocados
- 1 lime, squeezed for the juice
- 1 tbsp. extra-virgin olive oil
- 1 tbsp. fresh minced cilantro
- 1 diced small red onion
- 1 minced garlic clove
- Himalayan sea salt to taste
- black pepper, freshly ground

Brussels sprout:

- 3 lbs. of Brussels Sprout
- 1/2 cup raw honey
- 1/2 cup balsamic vinegar
- 1/2 cup melted coconut oil

- 1 cup dried cranberries
- Himalayan sea salt
- black pepper, freshly ground

Instructions:

To make the salmon and avocado sauce:

1. Combine cumin, onion, chili powder, garlic, and paprika seasoned with salt and pepper. Mix well before dry rubbing on the salmon.
2. Place the salmon in the fridge for 30 minutes.
3. Preheat the grill.
4. In a bowl, mash avocado until the texture becomes smooth. Pour in all the remaining ingredients and mix thoroughly.
5. Grill salmon for 5 minutes on each side or until cooked.
6. Drizzle avocado on cooked salmon.

To make the Brussel Sprout:

1. Preheat the oven to 375°F.
2. Mix Brussels Sprout with coconut oil. Season with salt and pepper.
3. Place vegetables on a baking sheet and roast for about 30 minutes.

4. In a separate pan, combine vinegar and honey.
5. Simmer in slow heat until it boils and thickens.
6. Drizzle them on top of the Brussels Sprouts.
7. Serve with the salmon.

Asian-Themed Macrobiotic Bowl

Ingredients:

- 2 cups cooked quinoa
- 4 carrots
- 1 package of smoked tofu
- 1 tbsp. nutritional yeast
- 2 tbsp. coconut aminos
- 4 tbsp. sunflower sprouts
- 2 tbsp. fermented vegetables
- 1 cup of shiitake mushrooms
- 1 avocado
- 2 tbsp. hemp seeds
- 2-3 cooked beets
- coconut oil cooking spray

Dressing:

- 2 tbsp. miso paste
- 1 tbsp. tahini
- 1 clove of garlic, crushed
- 1 tbsp. olive oil
- 1/2 lime, juiced
- 3 tbsp. water

Instructions:

1. Roast the carrots in the oven at 400°F for 30-40 minutes.

2. Wash the vegetables, trim, and spray them with coconut oil.
3. Add them to the oven. When they are cooked, set them aside till you are ready to assemble the Buddha bowl.
4. Make the dressing by combining all of the ingredients in a medium-size bowl. If the dressing appears lumpy, add more water.
5. To build the bowl, put the quinoa on the bottom and then arrange the vegetables on top.
6. Sprinkle the bowls with hemp seeds and drizzle the dressing over top.
7. Now serve and enjoy!

Chicken Salad

Ingredients:

- 1 small can of premium chunk chicken breast packed in water
- 1 stalk celery, large, finely chopped
- 1/4 cup reduced-fat mayonnaise
- 4 romaine leaves or red leaf lettuce, washed and trimmed
- 8 pcs. cherry tomatoes or 1 ripe tomato, quartered
- 1 cucumber, small and sliced thinly

Instructions:

1. Drain canned chicken and transfer to a bowl.
2. Put in celery and mayonnaise.
3. Mix lightly. Don't crush the chicken.
4. In a separate shallow bowl, place the lettuce neatly.
5. Add the chicken salad in the middle
6. Add tomatoes and cucumber slices to the plate.
7. Refrigerate before serving, cover with plastic wrap.

Baked Salmon

Ingredients:

- 2 salmon fillets
- 6 cups of fresh spinach
- 2 tsp. coconut oil
- 1/4 tsp. garlic powder
- 1/4 tsp. turmeric
- 3 large cloves of garlic
- lemon juice
- salt
- pepper

Instructions:

1. Preheat the oven to 400°F.
2. Line a baking dish with parchment paper.
3. Marinate salmon fillets in lemon juice, coconut oil, garlic powder, turmeric, salt, and pepper.
4. Let it sit for a few minutes. This may also be done the night before to help the juices and flavor get into the salmon.
5. Once the oven is ready, bake salmon for 15 minutes.
6. Cook some of the garlic in a pan with coconut oil.
7. Add spinach and cook until ready. Season with salt and pepper to taste.
8. Take salmon out of the oven and put spinach beside it.
9. Serve and enjoy.

Asian Zucchini Salad

Ingredients:

- 1 medium zucchini, sliced thinly into spirals
- 1/3 cup rice vinegar
- 3/4 cup avocado oil
- 1 cup sunflower seeds, shells removed
- 1 lb. cabbage, shredded
- 1 tsp. stevia drops
- 1 cup almonds, sliced

Instructions:

1. Cut the zucchini spirals into smaller parts. Set aside.
2. Put almonds, sunflower seeds, and cabbage in a large bowl. Combine the ingredients well.
3. Add zucchini to the mixture.
4. In a small bowl, mix vinegar, stevia, and oil using a whisk or fork.
5. Pour vinegar mixture all over the zucchini mixture. Toss well. Make sure everything is covered with the dressing.
6. Refrigerate for 2 hours before serving.

Low FODMAP Burger

Ingredients:

- 1-1/4 lbs. ground pork
- 1/4 tsp. allspice
- 1/2 tsp. salt
- 1/2 tsp. white pepper
- 1/2 tsp. ground nutmeg
- 1/2 tsp. caraway seeds
- 1/2 tsp. ground ginger

Instructions:

1. Preheat the grill then prepare the patty.
2. Using a small mixing bowl, stir together the salt, pepper, allspice, nutmeg, and ginger until fully combined.
3. Place the ground in a large mixing bowl and add the spice mixture.
4. Mix thoroughly until spices are evenly distributed to the pork.
5. Make round, flat burger patties using the palm of your hands.
6. Grill the patties and serve with gluten-free buns and mustard sauce.

Stir-Fried Cabbage and Apples

Ingredients:

- 1 shallot, thinly sliced
- 1/2 apple, cut into cubes
- 1/4 savoy cabbage, sliced thinly into strips
- 3–4 radishes, sliced thinly
- 1/2–1 tsp. coconut oil
- salt, to taste

Instructions:

1. Pour some coconut oil into a wok.
2. Add shallot and cook until translucent.
3. Add the cabbage, radish, and apples to the wok.
4. Stir-fry for about 5 minutes. Don't overcook.
5. Add salt to taste.
6. Serve while warm.

Asparagus and Greens Salad with Tahini and Poppy Seed Dressing

Ingredients:

- 10 to 12 asparagus stalks, washed well and sliced into ribbons
- 5 radishes, washed well and sliced thinly
- 2 to 3 rainbow carrots, peeled and sliced thinly
- 1 handful of wild spinach
- 1 small handful of microgreens, washed well
- 1 small handful of sunflower greens, washed well
- optional: a few pieces of chive blossoms

For the dressing:

- 2 tbsp. tahini
- 1 tbsp. poppy seeds
- 1 tbsp. extra-virgin olive oil
- salt
- pepper

Instructions:

1. For the dressing, whisk ingredients together in a small bowl.
2. In a separate bowl, toss salad ingredients into the mixture.
3. Drizzle dressing on salad upon serving.

Stir-Fried Cabbage and Apples

Ingredients:

- 1 shallot, thinly sliced
- 1/2 apple, cut into cubes
- 1/4 savoy cabbage, sliced thinly into strips
- 3–4 radishes, sliced thinly
- 1/2–1 tsp. coconut oil
- salt, to taste

Instructions:

1. Pour some coconut oil into a wok.
2. Add shallot and cook until translucent.
3. Add the cabbage, radish, and apples to the wok.
4. Stir-fry for about 5 minutes. Don't overcook.
5. Add salt to taste.
6. Serve while warm.

Roasted Chicken Thighs

Ingredients:

- 12 garlic cloves, unpeeled
- 1 tbsp. avocado oil
- 1 pinch Himalayan pink salt
- 4 chicken thighs with skin
- 1 tsp. Primal Palate super gyro seasoning

Instructions:

1. Pour avocado oil over a medium-sized oven-safe pot.
2. Add the garlic cloves. Sauté over medium heat for 2 to 3 minutes or until the skins begin to brown.
3. Place the chicken in a large skillet over medium-high heat. Sear for about 2 to 3 minutes for each side, starting with the skin side.
4. Combine the chicken with the garlic. Season generously with salt and Primal Palate Super Gyro seasoning.
5. Place the chicken in an oven preheated to 350°F.
6. Bake for one hour while covered.
7. Serve and enjoy.

Arugula and Mushroom Salad

Ingredients:

- 5 oz. arugula washed
- 1 lb. fresh mushrooms
- 1/4 tsp. shoyu
- 1/2 red onion
- 1 tbsp. olive oil
- 1 tbsp. mirin

For tofu cheese:

- 1/8 cup umeboshi vinegar
- 1/2 firm tofu

Instructions:

1. In a bowl, add the rinsed tofu. Crumble and pour in vinegar.
2. In a separate bowl add shoyu, red onions, salt, olive oil, and mirin. 3. Mix to combine.
3. Add in the arugula and toss to combine with the dressing.
4. Serve and enjoy.

Cauliflower and Mushroom Bake

Ingredients:

- 3 cups cauliflower florets
- 1 cup fresh mushroom, chopped
- 1/2 cup red onion, chopped
- 1/3 cup green onion, chopped
- 2 garlic cloves, finely chopped
- 2 tsp. apple cider vinegar
- 2 tsp. lemon juice
- 1/2 tsp. salt
- 1/4 tsp. pepper
- 1 tbsp. olive oil

Instructions:

1. Preheat the oven to 350°F. Lightly grease a baking pan.
2. Combine red onion, cauliflower, olive oil, garlic, mushroom, apple cider vinegar, lemon juice, salt, and pepper in a bowl. Mix well.
3. Pour the mixture into the greased baking pan.
4. Place inside the oven and bake for 45 minutes. Stir.
5. When vegetables are golden brown and tender, remove them from the oven.
6. Garnish with green onions. Serve and enjoy.

Conclusion

So there you have it! A beginner's quick start guide to managing CRPS through diet!

Complex regional pain syndrome (CRPS) is a chronic pain condition that usually affects one arm or leg. It is characterized by intense burning pain, swelling, and changes in the skin. There is no cure for CRPS, but there are treatments that can help to relieve the pain.

By following a healthy diet and making some lifestyle changes, you can help to reduce your symptoms and improve your quality of life. If you are living with CRPS, talk to your doctor about the best treatment options for you. There is no cure for CRPS, but treatments can help to improve your quality of life.

This guide is for informational purposes only and is not intended to be a substitute for professional medical advice, diagnosis, or treatment. Always seek the advice of your physician or other qualified healthcare providers with any questions you may have regarding a medical condition. Never disregard professional medical advice or delay in seeking it because of something you have read on this website.

FAQ About Complex Regional Pain Syndrome

What is complex regional pain syndrome (CRPS)?

Complex regional pain syndrome (CRPS) is a chronic pain condition that usually affects one arm or leg. It is characterized by intense burning pain, swelling, and changes in the skin. There is no cure for CRPS, but there are treatments that can help to relieve the pain.

What causes complex regional pain syndrome?

The exact cause of CRPS is unknown. It is thought to be the result of a problem with the nervous system.

What are the symptoms of complex regional pain syndrome?

The main symptom of CRPS is an intense burning pain that is out of proportion to the injury. Other symptoms include swelling, changes in skin color and texture, and joint stiffness.

How is complex regional pain syndrome diagnosed?

No one test can diagnose CRPS. The diagnosis is based on the symptoms and a physical examination.

What are the treatments for complex regional pain syndrome?

There is no cure for CRPS, but there are treatments that can help to relieve the pain. These include medication, physical therapy, and sympathetic nerve blocks.

Can complex regional pain syndrome be prevented?

There is no known way to prevent CRPS. However, early diagnosis and treatment may help to improve the symptoms.

What are some natural methods for managing CPRS?

Some natural methods that may help to relieve the pain of CRPS include acupuncture, massage, and meditation. Eating a healthy diet and getting regular exercise can also help.

References and Helpful Links

Can Diet Really Help CRPS and Chronic Pain? (2018, May 7). BLB Chronic Pain. https://www.blbchronicpain.co.uk/news/can-diet-really-help-crps-and-chronic-pain/.

Complex Regional Pain Syndrome (CRPS). (n.d.). Division of Pain Medicine. Retrieved September 28, 2022, from https://med.stanford.edu/pain/about/chronic-pain/crps.html.

Complex Regional Pain Syndrome Fact Sheet | National Institute of Neurological Disorders and Stroke. (n.d.). Retrieved September 28, 2022, from https://www.ninds.nih.gov/complex-regional-pain-syndrome-fact-sheet.

Complex Regional Pain Syndrome. (2017, October 19). NHS.uk. https://www.nhs.uk/conditions/complex-regional-pain-syndrome/.

CRPS Diet. (2019, April 8). Glenn Gittelson TMJ. https://www.drglenngittelsontmj.com/crps-diet/.

Reflex Sympathetic Dystrophy (RSD) Syndrome. (n.d.). Retrieved September 28, 2022, from https://www.health.ny.gov/diseases/chronic/reflex_sympathetic/.

Think Twice About Eating That-CRPS and Diet | Rsdsa. (2016, February 16). https://rsds.org/crps-and-diet-guest/.